The Definitive Vegetarian Savory Cookbook

Super Easy Savory Vegetarian Recipes For Beginners

Riley Bloom

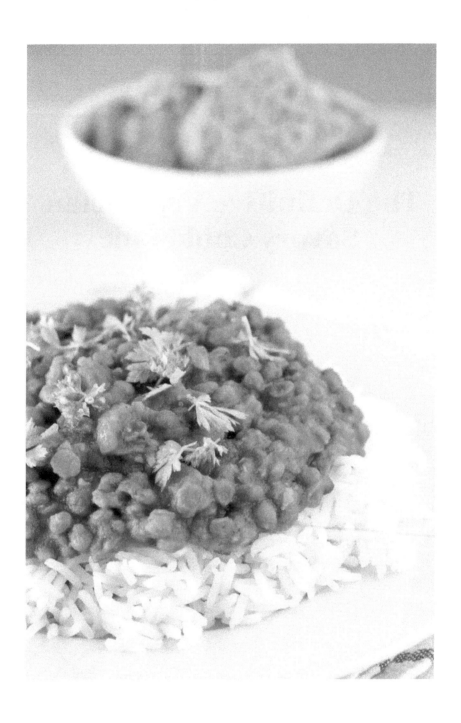

Table of contents

Simple Baked Spinach & Broccoli

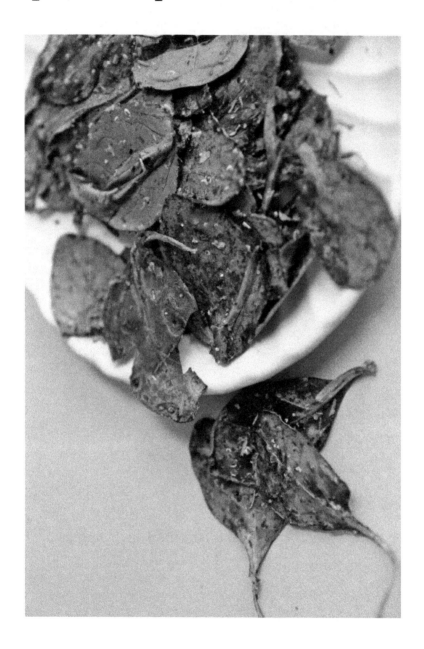

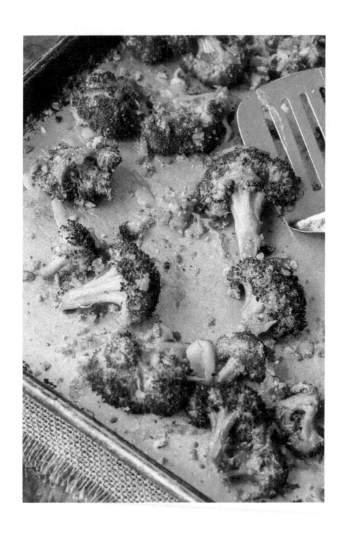

Ingredients

1 ½ pounds broccoli, peeled and cut into 1-inch chunks

½ red onion, thinly sliced

¼ cup vegetable stock

1 tbsp. extra virgin olive oil

½ tsp Italian seasoning

½ tsp hot chili powder

Black pepper

½ pound fresh spinach, roughly chopped

Directions:

Put all of the ingredients in a slow cooker except the last one. Top with handfuls of spinach and stuff the slow cooker with it. If you can't fit it all in at once, let the first batch cook first and add some more spinach. Cook for 3or 4 hours on medium until broccoli become soft. Scrape the sides and serve.

Roasted Endives and Brussels Sprouts

Ingredients

1 ½ pounds brussel sprouts, peeled and cut into 1-inch chunks

½ red onion, thinly sliced

¼ cup water

½ vegetable stock cube, crumbled

1 tbsp. extra virgin olive oil

½ tsp hot chili powder

Black pepper

½ pound endives, roughly chopped

Directions:

Put all of the ingredients in a slow cooker except the last one. Top with handfuls of endives and stuff the slow cooker with it. If you can't fit it all in at once, let the first batch cook first and add some more endives. Cook for 3 hours on medium until brussel sprouts become soft. Scrape the sides and serve.

Curried Sweet Potatoes and Swiss Chard

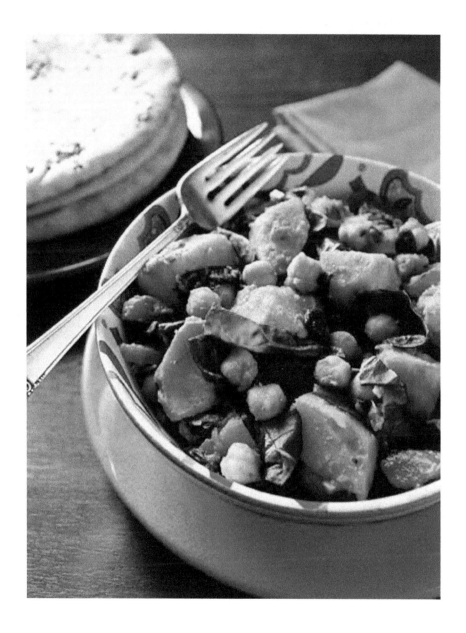

Ingredients

1 ½ pounds sweet potatoes, peeled and cut into 1-inch chunks

½ onion, thinly sliced

¼ cup water

½ vegetable stock cube, crumbled

1 tbsp. extra virgin olive oil

½ tsp cumin

½ tsp ground coriander

½ tsp garam masala

½ tsp hot chili powder

Black pepper

½ pound swiss chard, roughly chopped

Directions:

Put all of the ingredients in a slow cooker except the last one. Top with handfuls of swiss chard and stuff the slow cooker with it. If you can't fit it all in at once, let the first batch cook first and add some more swiss chard. Cook for 3or 4 hours on medium until sweet potatoes become soft. Scrape the sides and serve.

Collard Greens and Broccoli in Chili Garlic Sauce

Ingredients

1 ½ pounds carrots, peeled and cut into 1-inch chunks

½ pound broccoli, peeled and cut into 1-inch chunks

½ onion, thinly sliced

¼ cup water

½ vegetable stock cube, crumbled

1 tbsp. sesame oil

½ tsp chili garlic sauce

½ tsp. lime juice

½ tsp. minced green onions

Black pepper

½ pound collard greens, roughly chopped

Directions:

Put all of the ingredients in a slow cooker except the last one. Top with handfuls of collard greens and stuff the slow cooker with it. If you can't fit it all in at once, let the first batch cook first and add some more collard greens. Cook for 3or 4 hours on medium until carrots become soft. Scrape the sides and serve.

Mustard Greens and Shitake Mushroom

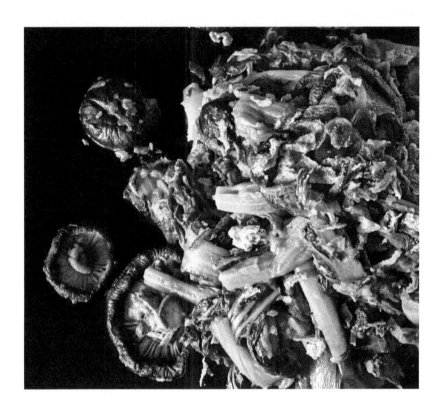

Ingredients

1 ½ pounds cauliflower, peeled and cut into 1-inch chunks

½ pound shitake mushrooms, sliced

½ red onion, thinly sliced

¼ cup vegetable stock

2 tbsp. sesame seed oil

½ tsp vinegar

½ tsp garlic, minced

Black pepper

½ pound fresh mustard greens, roughly chopped

Directions:

Put all of the ingredients in a slow cooker except the last one. Top with handfuls of mustard greens and stuff the slow cooker with it. If you can't fit it all in at once, let the first batch cook first and add some more mustard greens. Cook for 3 or 4 hours on medium until cauliflower become soft. Scrape the sides and serve.

Curried Rutabaga and Collard Greens

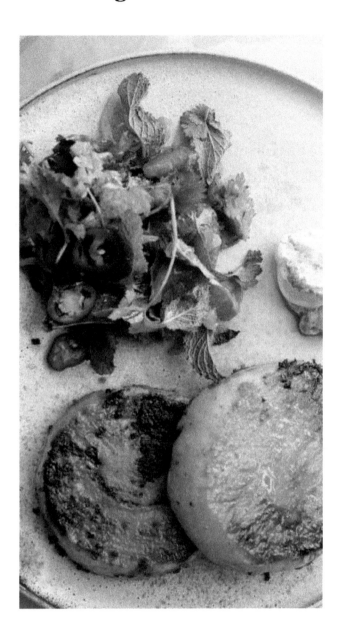

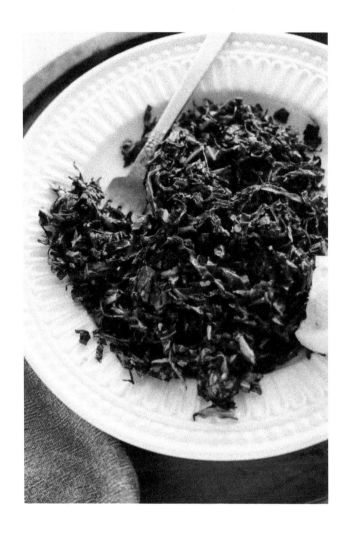

Ingredients

1 ½ pounds rutabaga , peeled and cut into 1-inch chunks

½ onion, thinly sliced

¼ cup vegetable stock

1 tbsp. extra virgin olive oil

2 tbsp. red curry powder

Black pepper

½ pound fresh collard greens, roughly chopped

Directions:

Put all of the ingredients in a slow cooker except the last one. Top with handfuls of collard greens and stuff the slow cooker with it. If you can't fit it all in at once, let the first batch cook first and add some more collard greens. Cook for 3 or 4 hours on medium until rutabaga become soft. Scrape the sides and serve.

Swiss Chard and Yam in Pesto Sauce

Ingredients

1 ½ pounds yam, peeled and cut into 1-inch chunks

½ red onion, thinly sliced

¼ cup vegetable stock

2 tbsp. extra virgin olive oil

3 tbsp. pesto sauce

Black pepper

½ pound fresh Swiss Chard, roughly chopped

Directions:

Put all of the ingredients in a slow cooker except the last one. Top with handfuls of Swiss Chard and stuff the slow cooker with it. If you can't fit it all in at once, let the first batch cook first and add some more Swiss Chard. Cook for 3 or 4 hours on medium until yam become soft. Scrape the sides and serve.

Slow Cooked Turnip Greens and Butternut Squash

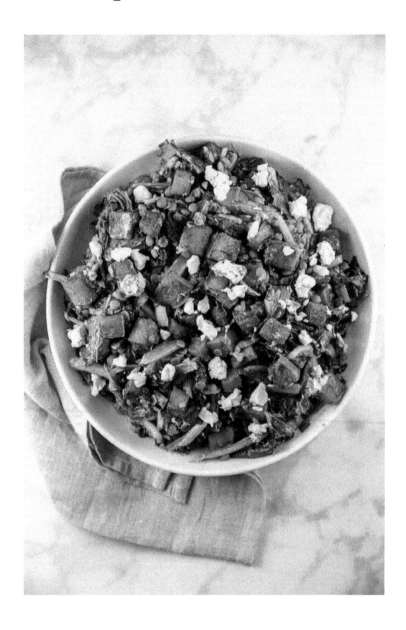

Ingredients

1 ½ pounds butternut squash, peeled and cut into 1-inch chunks

½ onion, thinly sliced

¼ cup vegetable stock

1 tbsp. extra virgin olive oil

Black pepper

½ pound fresh Turnip greens, roughly chopped

Directions:

Put all of the ingredients in a slow cooker except the last one. Top with handfuls of spinach and stuff the slow cooker with it. If you can't fit it all in at once, let the first batch cook first and add some more spinach. Cook for 3or 4 hours on medium until butternut squash become soft. Scrape the sides and serve.

Slow Cooked Endives and Winter Squash in Pesto Sauce

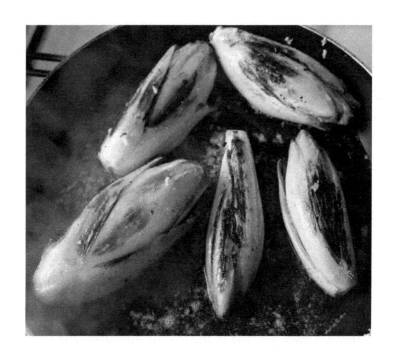

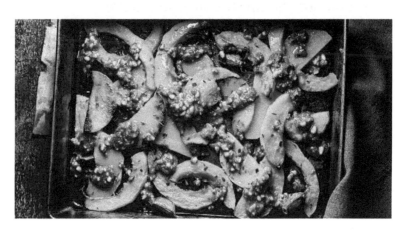

Ingredients

1 ½ pounds winter squash, peeled and cut into 1-inch chunks

½ onion, thinly sliced

¼ cup vegetable stock

1 tbsp. extra virgin olive oil

2 tbsp. pesto sauce

Black pepper

½ pound fresh Endive, roughly chopped

Directions:

Put all of the ingredients in a slow cooker except the last one. Top with handfuls of endive and stuff the slow cooker with it. If you can't fit it all in at once, let the first batch cook first and add some more endive. Cook for 3or 4 hours on medium until winter squash become soft. Scrape the sides and serve.

Slow-cooked Microgreens and Potatoes

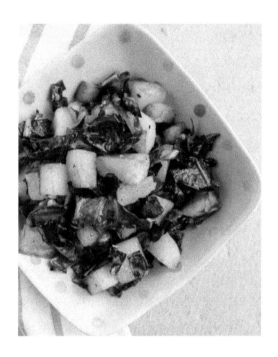

Ingredients

1 ½ pounds potatoes, peeled and cut into 1-inch chunks

½ onion, thinly sliced

¼ cup vegetable stock

1 tbsp. extra virgin olive oil

1 tsp. Italian seasoning

Black pepper

½ pound microgreens, roughly chopped

Directions:

Put all of the ingredients in a slow cooker except the last one. Top with handfuls of microgreens and stuff the slow cooker with it. If you can't fit it all in at once, let the first batch cook first and add some more microgreens. Cook for 3or 4 hours on medium until potatoes become soft. Scrape the sides and serve.

Buttery Watercress and Parsnips

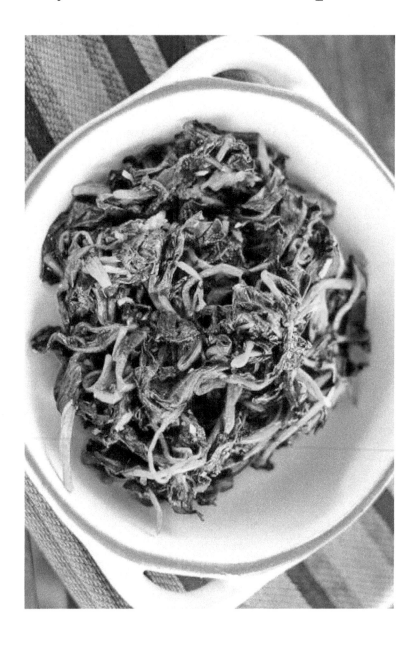

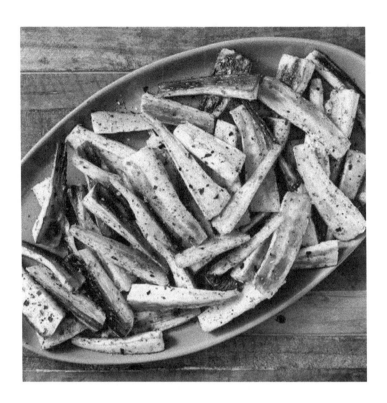

Ingredients

1 ½ pounds parsnips, peeled and cut into 1-inch chunks

½ onion, thinly sliced

¼ cup vegetable stock

4 tbsp. melted vegan butter

2 tbsp. lemon juice

Black pepper

½ pound fresh Watercress, roughly chopped

Directions:

Put all of the ingredients in a slow cooker except the last one. Top with handfuls of watercress and stuff the slow cooker with it. If you can't fit it all in at once, let the first batch cook first and add some more Watercress. Cook for 3or 4 hours on medium until parsnips become soft. Scrape the sides and serve.

Slow Cooked Bok Choy and Carrots

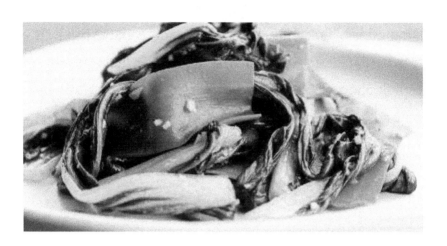

Ingredients

1 ½ pounds carrots, peeled and cut into 1-inch chunks

½ onion, thinly sliced

¼ cup vegetable stock

1 tbsp. sesame oil

1 tbsp. canola oil

2 tbsp. hoi sin sauce

Black pepper

½ pound fresh Bok Choy, roughly chopped

Directions:

Put all of the ingredients in a slow cooker except the last one. Top with handfuls of bok choy and stuff the slow cooker with it. If you can't fit it all in at once, let the first batch cook first and add some more bok choy. Cook for 3or 4 hours on medium until carrots become soft. Scrape the sides and serve.

Slow Cooked Mustard Greens and Sweet Potatoes

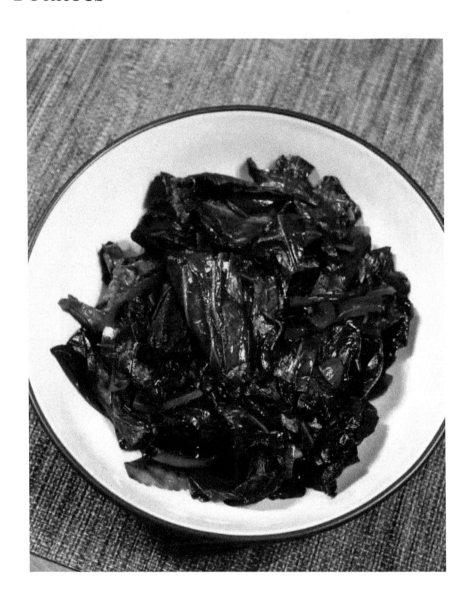

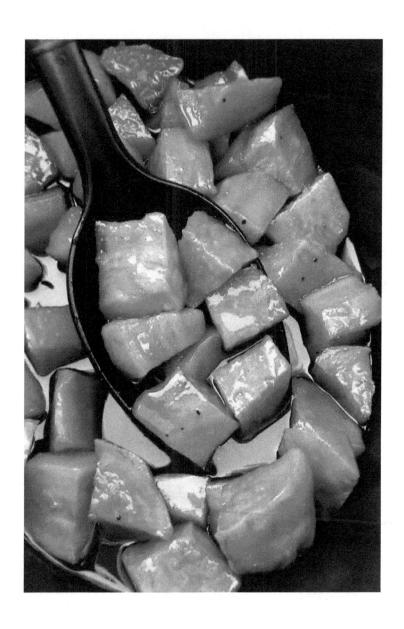

Ingredients

1 ½ pounds sweet potatoes, peeled and cut into 1-inch chunks

½ onion, thinly sliced

¼ cup vegetable stock

1 tbsp. extra virgin olive oil

2 tbsp. pesto sauce

Black pepper

½ pound fresh mustard greens, roughly chopped

Directions:

Put all of the ingredients in a slow cooker except the last one. Top with handfuls of mustard greens and stuff the slow cooker with it. If you can't fit it all in at once, let the first batch cook first and add some more mustard greens. Cook for 3or 4 hours on medium until sweet potatoes become soft. Scrape the sides and serve.

Slow Cooked Cabbage and Rutabaga

Ingredients

1 ½ pounds rutabaga, peeled and cut into 1-inch chunks

½ onion, thinly sliced

¼ cup vegetable stock

1 tbsp. extra virgin olive oil

Black pepper

½ pound fresh cabbage, roughly chopped

Directions:

Put all of the ingredients in a slow cooker except the last one. Top with handfuls of cabbage and stuff the slow cooker with it. If you can't fit it all in at once, let the first batch cook first and add some more cabbage. Cook for 3or 4 hours on medium until carrots become soft. Scrape the sides and serve.

Slow Cooked Turnip Greens & Yam

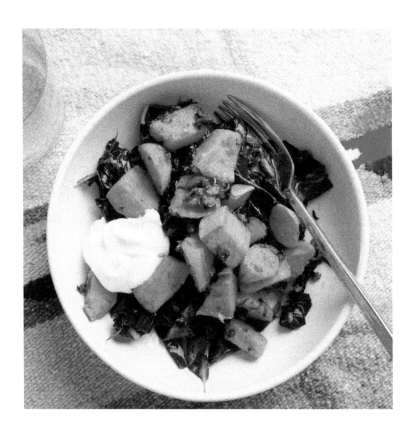

Ingredients

1 ½ pounds yam, peeled and cut into 1-inch chunks

½ onion, thinly sliced

¼ cup vegetable stock

1 tbsp. extra virgin olive oil

2 tbsp. pesto sauce

Black pepper

½ pound fresh turnip greens, roughly chopped

Directions:

Put all of the ingredients in a slow cooker except the last one. Top with handfuls of turnip greens and stuff the slow cooker with it. If you can't fit it all in at once, let the first batch cook first and add some more turnip greens. Cook for 3or 4 hours on medium until yam become soft. Scrape the sides and serve.

Slow Cooked Mustard Greens & Potatoes in Pesto Sauce

Ingredients

1 ½ pounds potatoes, peeled and cut into 1-inch chunks

½ onion, thinly sliced

¼ cup vegetable stock

1 tbsp. extra virgin olive oil

2 tbsp. pesto sauce

Black pepper

½ pound fresh mustard greens, roughly chopped

Directions:

Put all of the ingredients in a slow cooker except the last one. Top with handfuls of mustard greens and stuff the slow cooker with it. If you can't fit it all in at once, let the first batch cook first and add some more mustard greens. Cook for 3 or 4 hours on medium until potatoes become soft. Scrape the sides and serve.

Buttery Oyster Mushrooms and Kale

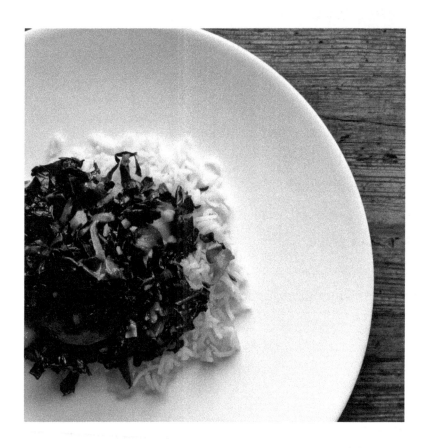

Ingredients

1 ½ pounds oyster mushrooms

½ onion, thinly sliced

¼ cup vegetable stock

2 tbsp. vegan butter or margarine

1 tsp. herbs de Provence

Black pepper

½ pound fresh kale, roughly chopped

Directions:

Put all of the ingredients in a slow cooker except the last one. Top with handfuls of kale and stuff the slow cooker with it. If you can't fit it all in at once, let the first batch cook first and add some more kale. Cook for 3or 4 hours on medium until mushrooms become soft. Scrape the sides and serve.

Slow cooked Italian-style Swiss Chard

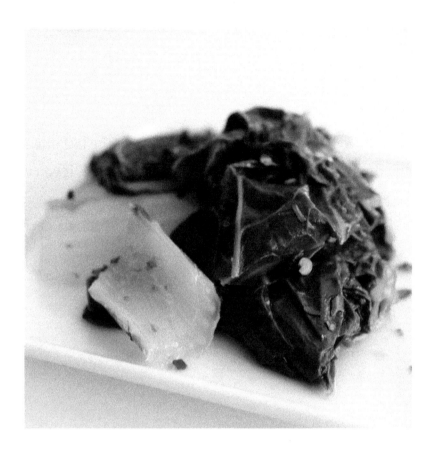

Ingredients

1 ½ pounds crimini mushrooms

½ onion, thinly sliced

¼ cup vegetable stock

1 tbsp. extra virgin olive oil

2 tbsp. garlic

1 tsp. Italian seasoning

Black pepper

½ pound fresh swiss chard, roughly chopped

Directions:

Put all of the ingredients in a slow cooker except the last one. Top with handfuls of swiss chard and stuff the slow cooker with it. If you can't fit it all in at once, let the first batch cook first and add some more swiss chard. Cook for 3 or 4 hours on medium until mushrooms become soft. Scrape the sides and serve.

Slow Cooked Oyster Mushrooms and Spinach in Yellow Bean Sauce

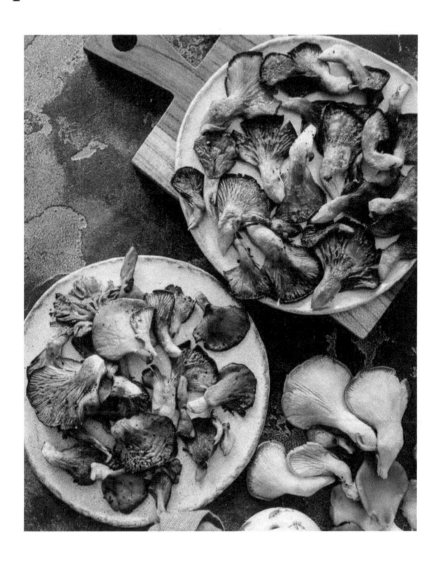

Ingredients

1 ½ pounds oyster mushrooms

½ onion, thinly sliced

¼ cup vegetable stock

1 tbsp. sesame oil

2 tbsp. yellow bean sauce

Black pepper

½ pound fresh spinach, roughly chopped

Directions:

Put all of the ingredients in a slow cooker except the last one. Top with handfuls of spinach and stuff the slow cooker with it. If you can't fit it all in at once, let the first batch cook first and add some more spinach. Cook for 3or 4 hours on medium until mushrooms become soft. Scrape the sides and serve.

Slow Cooked Sichuan Style Watercress & Enoki Mushrooms

Ingredients

1 ½ pounds enoki mushrooms

½ onion, thinly sliced

¼ cup vegetable stock

1 tbsp. sesame oil

1 tsp. Sichuan peppercorn

Black pepper

½ pound fresh watercress, roughly chopped

Directions:

Put all of the ingredients in a slow cooker except the last one. Top with handfuls of watercress and stuff the slow cooker with it. If you can't fit it all in at once, let the first batch cook first and add some more watercress. Cook for 3or 4 hours on medium until mushrooms become soft. Scrape the sides and serve.

Slow Cooked thai Style Turnip Greens and Chanterelle Mushrooms

Ingredients

1 ½ pounds chanterelle mushrooms

½ onion, thinly sliced

¼ cup vegetable stock

2 tbsp. sesame oil

2 tbsp. Thai chili garlic paste

2 leaves

Thai Basil

Black pepper

½ pound fresh turnip greens, roughly chopped

Directions:

Put all of the ingredients in a slow cooker except the last one. Top with handfuls of turnip greens and stuff the slow cooker with it. If you can't fit it all in at once, let the first batch cook first and add some more turnip greens. Cook for 3or 4 hours on medium until mushrooms become soft. Scrape the sides and serve.

Slow Mustard Greens and Enoki Mushrooms

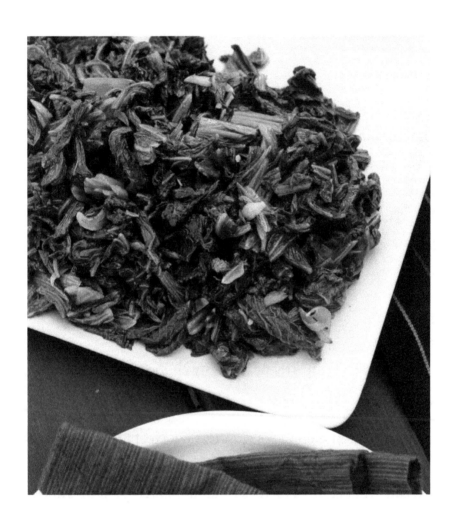

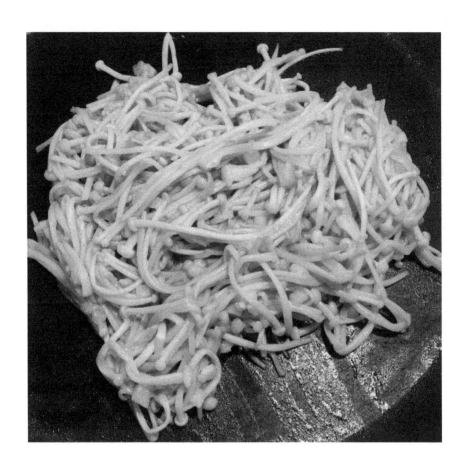

Ingredients

1 ½ pounds enoki mushrooms

½ onion, thinly sliced

¼ cup vegetable stock

1 tbsp. extra virgin olive oil

2 tbsp. olives

2 tbsp. capers

Black pepper

½ pound fresh mustard greens, roughly chopped

Directions:

Put all of the ingredients in a slow cooker except the last one. Top with handfuls of mustard greens and stuff the slow cooker with it. If you can't fit it all in at once, let the first batch cook first and add some more mustard greens. Cook for 3or 4 hours on medium until mushrooms become soft. Scrape the sides and serve.

Slow cooked Choy Sum and Shitake Mushrooms

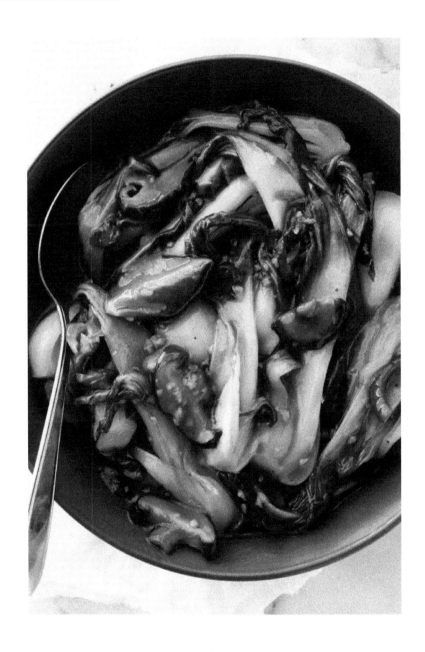

Ingredients

1 ½ pounds shitake mushrooms

½ onion, thinly sliced

¼ cup vegetable stock

2 tbsp. sesame seed oil

1 tbsp. hoi sin sauce

1 tbsp. hoi sin sauce

Black pepper

½ pound fresh choy sum, roughly chopped

Directions:

Put all of the ingredients in a slow cooker except the last one. Top with handfuls of choy sum and stuff the slow cooker with it. If you can't fit it all in at once, let the first batch cook first and add some more choy sum. Cook for 3or 4 hours on medium until mushrooms become soft. Scrape the sides and serve.

Slow Cooked Mustard Greens and Porcini Mushrooms

Ingredients

1 ½ pounds porcini mushrooms

½ onion, thinly sliced

¼ cup vegetable stock

1 tbsp. melted vegan butter

1 tbsp. garlic powder

1 tbsp. lime

Black pepper

½ pound mustard greens, roughly chopped

Directions:

Put all of the ingredients in a slow cooker except the last one. Top with handfuls of mustard greens and stuff the slow cooker with it. If you can't fit it all in at once, let the first batch cook first and add some more mustard greens. Cook for 3or 4 hours on medium until mushrooms become soft. Scrape the sides and serve.

Slow Cooked Turnip Greens and Enoki Mushrooms in Yellow Bean Sauce

Ingredients

1 ½ pounds enoki mushrooms

½ onion, thinly sliced

¼ cup vegetable stock

1 tbsp. sesame oil

2 tbsp. yellow bean sauce

Black pepper

½ pound fresh turnip greens, roughly chopped

Directions:

Put all of the ingredients in a slow cooker except the last one. Top with handfuls of turnip greens and stuff the slow cooker with it. If you can't fit it all in at once, let the first batch cook first and add some more turnip greens. Cook for 3or 4 hours on medium until mushrooms become soft. Scrape the sides and serve.

Lentils and Sweet Potato Curry

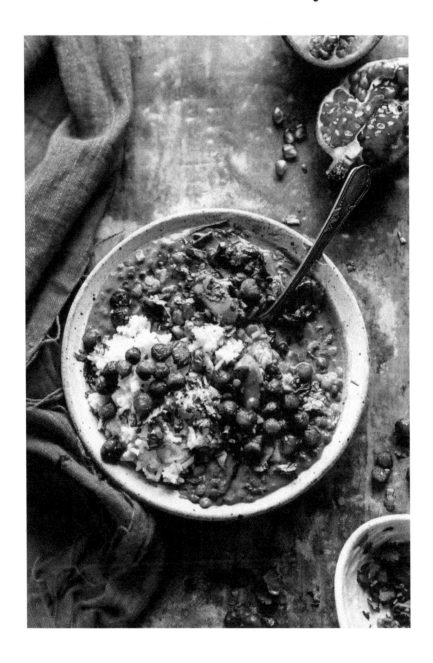

Ingredients

3 large sweet potatoes, diced (about 6 cups)

3 cups vegetable stock

1 red onion, minced

6 cloves garlic, minced

2 teaspoon each ground coriander, garam masala, and chili powder

1/2 teaspoon sea salt

1 1/2 cups uncooked red lentils (masoor dal)

1 can coconut milk

1 cup water

combine the sweet potatoes, vegetable stock, onion, garlic, and spices in a slow cooker.

Directions:

Cook on high heat in a slow cooker for 3 hours or until vegetables become soft. Add the lentils and combine. Cook on high for another hour and a half. Add the coconut milk. Add water as needed.

Slow Cooked Jambalaya

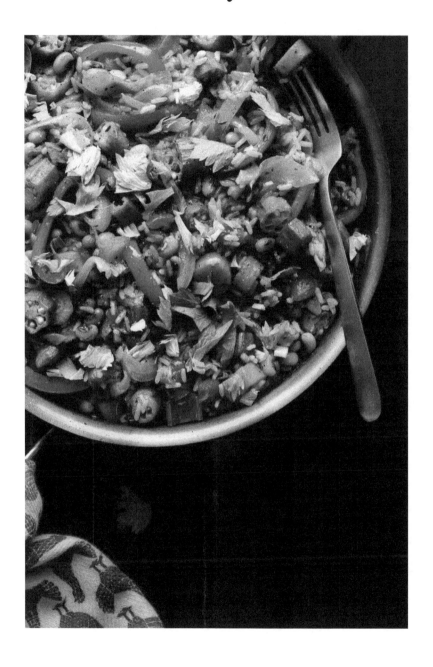

Ingredients

6 oz soy chorizo* (optional)

5 jalapeno peppers, diced

¾ cup okra,

½" inch rounds

½ red onion, diced

3 celery ribs (about 1½ cups)

4 cloves garlic, minced

1 16-oz can of Rotel (diced tomatoes & green chilies)

1½ cups vegetable stock

½ tsp paprika

¼ tsp sea salt

¼ tsp ground

Black pepper

½ tsp cayenne pepper

3 cups cooked cilantro rice

Directions:

Cook the soy chorizo on medium-high heat. Simmer and put in the Crockpot. Add the jalapeno pepper, red onion, celery, & garlic to the slow cooker. Add the diced tomatoes and vegetable stock. Add the seasoning and give the vegetables a nice stir.

Cook on low for 5 hours or on high for about 2 hours and 15 minutes. Add the cooked rice and stir with the rest of the ingredients in the slow cooker 30 minutes before serving.

Baked Baby Potatoes and Green Beans

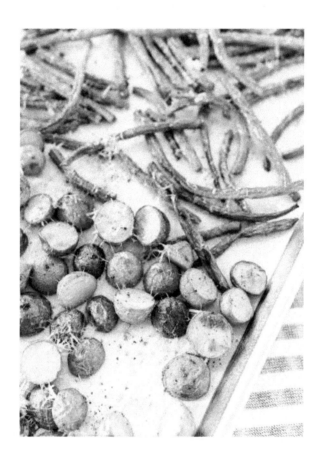

Ingredients

2 cups baby potatoes

3 tablespoons extra virgin olive oil, divided

2 cups grape tomatoes

2 cups 1-inch cut fresh green beans

6 cloves garlic, minced

2 teaspoons dried basil

1 teaspoon sea salt

1 (15 ounce) can chick peas, drained and rinsed

2 teaspoons extra virgin olive oil, or to taste (optional)

Sea salt Ground

Black pepper to taste

Directions:

Preheat your oven to 425 degrees F. Cover the baking pan with aluminum foil. Coat the potatoes with 1 tablespoon olive oil in a bowl. Pour into the pan and roast in the oven until tender, for half an hour. Add the tomatoes, beans, garlic, basil, and Sea salt with 2 tablespoons olive oil. Take the potatoes out of the oven and move them to one side of the pan. Add the tomato and green beans. Roast until tomatoes begin to wilt for 18 minutes more. Take it out of the oven and pour into a dish. Add garbanzo beans, 2 teaspoons olive oil, salt and pepper.

Baked Lima Beans Summer Squash & Potatoes

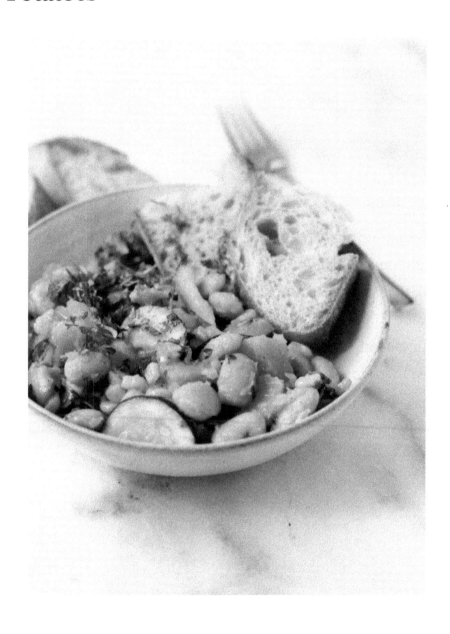

Ingredients

2 (15 ounce) cans lima beans, rinsed and drained

1/2 summer squash - peeled, seeded, and cut into 1-inch pieces

1 red onion, diced

2 large carrots, cut into 1 inch pieces

4 medium russet potatoes, cut into 1-inch pieces

3 tablespoons olive oil

1 teaspoon Sea salt

1/2 teaspoon ground

Black pepper

1 teaspoon onion powder

1 teaspoon garlic powder

1 teaspoon ground fennel seeds

1 teaspoon dried rubbed sage

2 green scallions, chopped (optional)

Directions:

Preheat your oven to 350 degrees F. Layer the beans, summer squash, onion, sweet potato, carrots, and russet potatoes on an oiled pan. Drizzle with olive oil and coat. Mix the salt, black pepper, onion powder, garlic powder, ground fennel seeds, and rubbed sage thoroughly in a bowl. Sprinkle this seasoning over vegetables on a pan.

Bake in the oven for 25 minutes. Roast until vegetables are soft and lightly browned, for around 23 minutes. Season with more salt and pepper to taste Sprinkle with chopped green onion.

Baked Green Beans and Sweet Potatoes

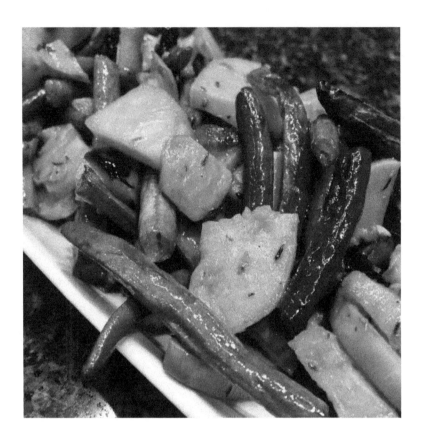

Ingredients

1 1/2 pounds sweet potatoes, cut into chunks

2 tablespoons extra virgin olive oil

8 cloves garlic, thinly sliced

4 teaspoons dried rosemary

4 teaspoons dried thyme

2 teaspoons

Sea salt

1 bunch fresh green beans, trimmed and cut into 1 inch pieces

ground Black pepper to taste

Directions:

Preheat your oven to 425 degrees F Combine the potatoes with 1 tbsp. of olive oil, garlic, rosemary, thyme, and 1 tsp. sea salt. Wrap with aluminum foil. Roast for 20 minutes in the oven. Combine the green beans, remaining olive oil, and remaining salt. Cover, and cook for another 15 minutes, until the potatoes are tender. Increase your oven temperature to 450 degrees F. Take out the foil, and cook for 8 minutes, until potatoes are browned. Sprinkle with pepper.

Baked Crimini Mushrooms and Cherry Tomatoes

Ingredients

1 pound potatoes, halved

2 tablespoons extra virgin olive oil

1/2 pound cremini mushrooms

8 cloves unpeeled garlic

2 tablespoons chopped fresh thyme

1 tablespoon olive oil

Sea salt ground

Black pepper to taste

1/4 pound cherry tomatoes

3 tablespoons toasted pine nuts

1/4 pound spinach, thinly sliced

Directions:

Preheat your oven to 425 degrees F. Place the potatoes on a baking pan and drizzle with 2 tablespoons of olive oil. Roast for 15 minutes and turn it once. Add the mushrooms, with the stem sides up, and garlic cloves to pan. Sprinkle with thyme and 1 tablespoon olive oil Season with Sea salt and black pepper. Bring it back to the oven; cook 5 minutes. Add the tomatoes to the pan. Bake until mushrooms are softened for about 5 more minutes.

Sprinkle pine nuts over potatoes and mushrooms. Garnish with sliced spinach.

Vegan Winter Squash and Zucchini Fajitas

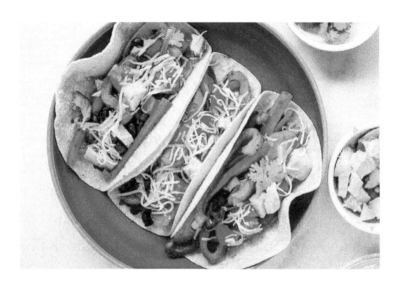

Ingredients

1/4 cup olive oil

1/4 cup red wine vinegar

A Pinch of dried oregano

1 teaspoon chili powder garlic

salt to taste salt and pepper to taste

1 teaspoon honey

2 small zucchini, julienned

2 medium winter squash, julienned

1 large red onion, sliced

5 jalapeno peppers, minced

2 tablespoons extra virgin olive oil

1 (8.75 ounce) can whole kernel corn, drained

1 (15 ounce) can pinto beans, drained

Directions:

Mix the olive oil, vinegar, oregano, chili powder, garlic salt, salt, pepper and honey thoroughly. To this marinade add the zucchini, squash, red onion, and jalapeno peppers. Marinate in the refrigerator for an hour or overnight. Heat the olive oil over medium-high heat. Drain the vegetables and sauté until tender for about 12 minutes. Add the corn and beans. Increase the heat to high until you brown the vegetables.

Easy Steamed Asparagus

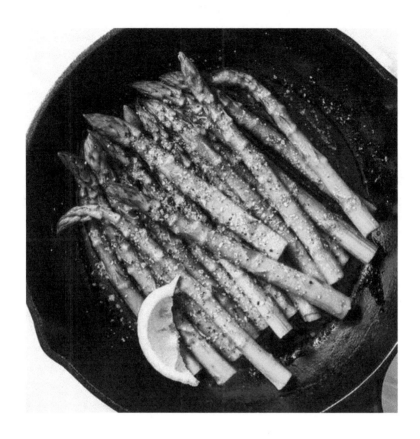

Ingredients

1 bunch asparagus spears

1 teaspoon extra virgin olive oil

1/4 teaspoon

Sea salt

3 cups water

Place water in the bottom half of a steamer pan set. Add salt and oil, and bring to a boil.

Directions:

Trim the dry ends off of the asparagus. If the spears are thick, peel them lightly with a vegetable peeler. Place them in the top half of the steamer pan set. Steam for 5 to 10 minutes depending on the thickness of the asparagus, or until asparagus is tender.

Chinese Style Steamed Choy Sum

Ingredients

1 bunch choy sum

1 teaspoon sesame seed oil

1/4 teaspoon

Sea salt

3 cups water

Directions:

Place water in the bottom half of a steamer pan set. Add salt and oil, and bring to a boil. Place the vegetable in the top half of the steamer pan set. Steam for 5 to 10 minutes depending on the thickness of the vegetable, or until vegetable becomes tender.

Easy Steamed Spinach

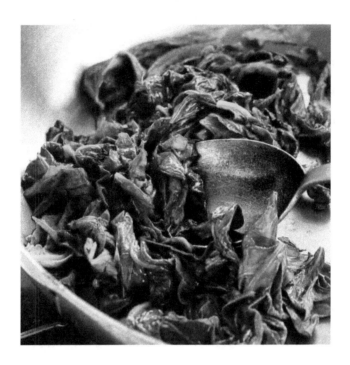

Ingredients

1 bunch Spinach

1 teaspoon extra virgin olive oil

1/4 teaspoon

Sea salt

3 cups water

Place water in the bottom half of a steamer pan set.

Add salt and oil, and bring to a boil.

Directions:

Place the vegetable in the top half of the steamer pan set. Steam for 5 to 10 minutes depending on the thickness of the vegetable, or until vegetable becomes tender.

Simple Steamed Watercress

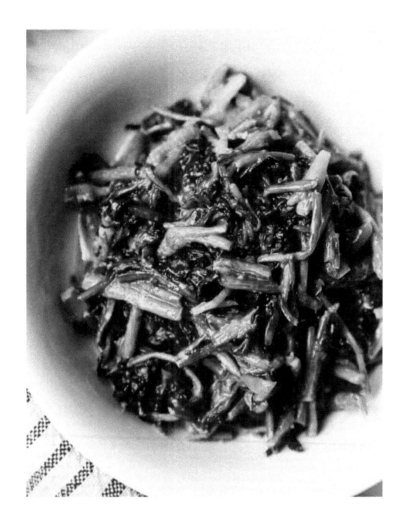

Ingredients

1 bunch watercress

1 teaspoon extra virgin olive oil

1/4 teaspoon

Sea salt

3 cups water

Directions:

Place water in the bottom half of a steamer pan set.
Add salt and oil, and bring to a boil. Place the vegetable in the
top half of the steamer pan set. Steam for 5 to 10 minutes
depending on the thickness of the vegetable, or until vegetable
becomes tender.

Vegetarian Pad Thai Sauce

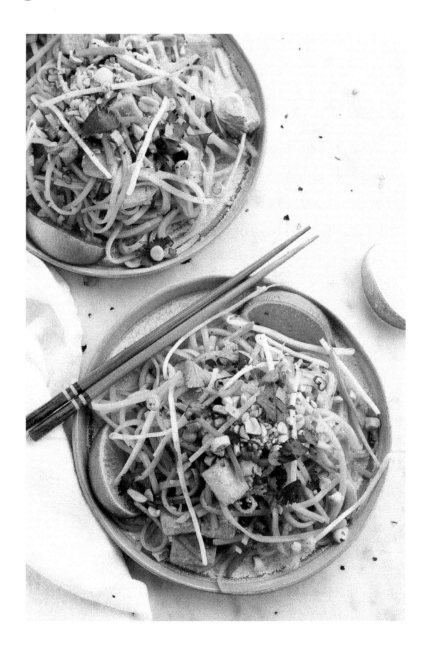

Ingredients

1/2 cup honey

1/2 cup distilled white vinegar

1/4 cup soy sauce

2 tablespoons tamarind pulp

Main Ingredients

1 (12 ounce) package dried rice noodles

1/2 cup sesame seed oil

2 teaspoons minced garlic

4 eggs

1 (12 ounce) package firm tofu, cut into 1/2 inch strips

1 tablespoon and 1 tsp. honey

1 1/2 teaspoons Sea salt

1 1/2 cups ground peanuts

1 1/2 teaspoons ground, dried

oriental radish 1/2 cup

chopped fresh chives 1 tablespoon

Directions:

Thai chili garlic paste 2 cups fresh bean sprouts 1 lime, cut into wedges Over medium heat combine all of the sauce ingredients Soak the rice noodles in cold water until soft and drain. In a large pan, warm the olive oil, garlic and eggs over medium heat. Stir to scramble the eggs. Add the tofu and stir Add the noodles and stir until cooked. Add the sauce, 1 1/2 tablespoons honey and 1 1/2 teaspoons sea salt. Add the peanuts and ground radish. Take it off the heat and add chives and chili garlic paste. Garnish with lime and bean sprouts.

Vegetarian Garbanzo Bean Sandwich Filling

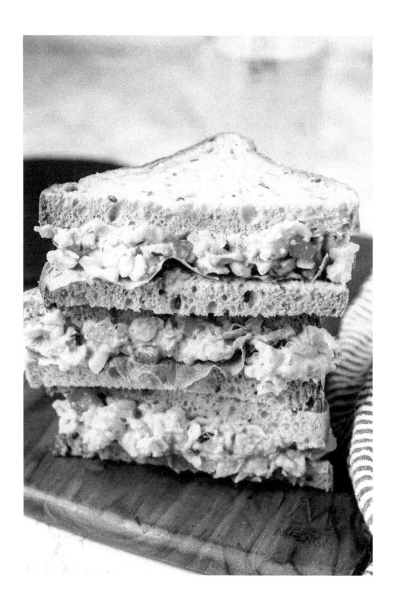

Ingredients

1 (19 ounce) can garbanzo beans, drained and rinsed

1 stalk celery, chopped

1/2 red onion, chopped

1 tablespoon mayonnaise

1 tablespoon lemon juice

1 teaspoon dried dill weed

Sea salt Pepper to taste

Directions:

Rinse and drain the beans. Pour the beans into a bowl and mash with a fork. Stir in celery, onion, vegan mayonnaise, lemon juice, dill, sea salt and pepper to taste.

Vegetarian Sloppy Joe

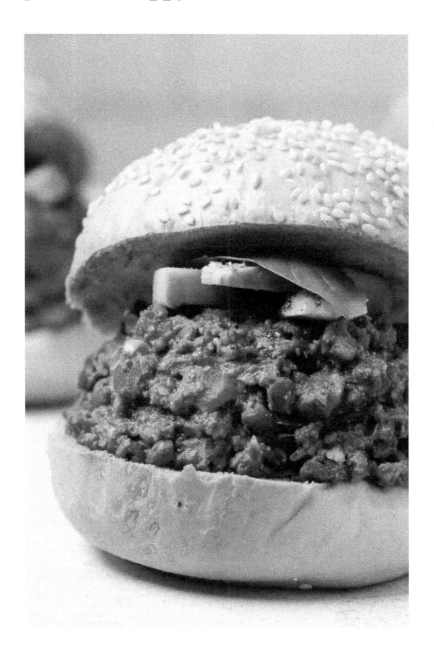

Ingredients

1 tablespoon oil, or as needed

1/2 red onion, minced

1/2 red bell pepper, minced

¼ cup minced garlic

1 cup water

3/4 cup ketchup

3 tablespoons spicy brown mustard

2 tablespoons soy sauce

2 tablespoons vegan barbeque sauce (ex. Simple Girl Organic)

1 tablespoon maple syrup

1 tablespoon Tabasco or Frank's hot sauce

1 teaspoon thyme

1 teaspoon cayenne pepper, or to taste

2 cups cooked garbanzo beans, or more to taste

Directions:

Heat oil in a pan over medium heat. Sauté the onion, red bell pepper, and garlic until tender for about 10 minutes. Add the water, ketchup, mustard, soy sauce, barbeque sauce, honey, hot sauce, thyme, and cayenne pepper to the mixture.

Boil this mixture. Reduce heat and simmer until sauce thickens, for about 5 minutes. Add the beans into the sauce and simmer until beans are warmed.

Vegetarian Quinoa and Chickpea Burger

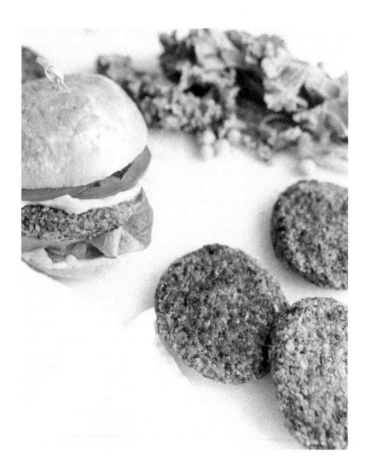

Ingredients

1 1/2 cups cooked quinoa

2 tablespoons Dijon mustard

1 egg vegan (Brand: Follow Your Heart Egg Vegan), beaten

2 cloves garlic, minced

2 grinds fresh Black pepper

1/2 cup chickpea (garbanzo bean) flour, or as needed

2 teaspoons olive oil, or as needed

2 slices gouda cheese

Combine the quinoa, mustard, vegan egg, garlic, and black pepper together in a bowl; add enough chickpea flour to make 2 patties.

Directions:

Heat oil in a pan over medium heat Cook patties in oil until browned for around 4 minutes per side. Add a vegan cheese slice to each patty and warm until cheese melts, about 2 and a half minutes.

Roasted Tofu in Chili Garlic Sauce

Ingredients

1 (18 ounce) package extra-firm tofu, slice

1/2-inch thick

2 tablespoons sesame oil

1 pinch Sea salt

1 pinch ground

Black pepper

2 tablespoons soy sauce

2 tablespoons Sriracha hot sauce, or to taste

1 1/2 teaspoons sesame oil

1 teaspoon chili-garlic sauce

1 teaspoon sesame seeds

1/2 teaspoon minced garlic

1 scallions, thinly sliced

Directions:

Preheat your oven to 450 degrees F. Layer the tofu slices onto a baking pan. Brush olive oil on each slice. Season salt and pepper over the tofu. Bake tofu in the oven until lightly browned, about 9 minutes. Add the soy sauce, Sriracha, sesame oil, chili garlic sauce, sesame seeds, garlic, and green onion Sprinkle on top of the tofu slices. Roast for 4 minutes more.

Vegetarian Reuben Sandwich

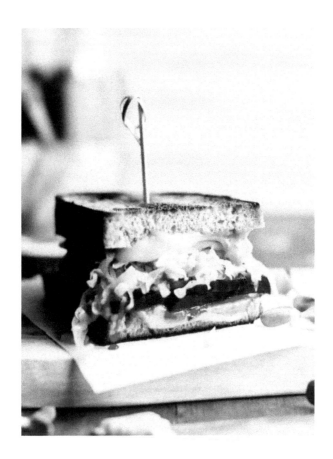

Ingredients

1 pound cheddar cheese, shredded

1 cup ranch salad dressing, or to taste

1 (16 ounce) jar sauerkraut, drained

12 slices dark rye bread

2 tablespoons olive oil

2 tomatoes, sliced

Directions:

Combine the cheese and sauerkraut thoroughly. Add the dressing and mix thoroughly. Brush each slice of bread with olive oil on one side. Spread a thick layer of the vegan cheese mixture onto unbuttered side of half of each bread. Top with tomato and another slice of bread. Heat a large pan to medium-high. Fry sandwiches on both sides until toasted and the cheese has melted.

Simple Deep-fried Jack Fruit

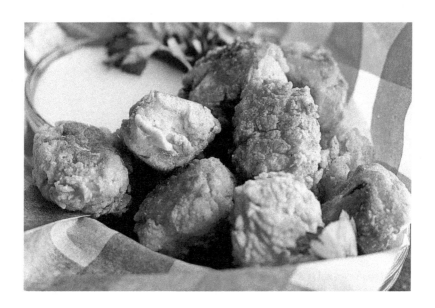

Ingredients

Drop of maple syrup

salt to taste

2 cups water oil for frying

10 pieces drained jackfruit

Dredging Mix

4 cups all-purpose flour

1/2 teaspoon ground turmeric

1/4 teaspoon baking powder

Directions:

Combine all of the dredging mix ingredients in a bowl. Add in water until batter becomes thick. Heat oil in a deep-fryer over medium heat. Dip jackfruit in the batter Cook in small batches in oil until golden brown, 2 to 3 minutes per side.

Simple Roasted Summer Squash

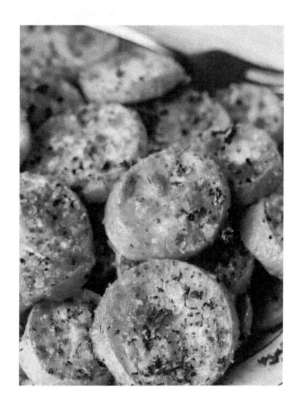

Ingredients

1 summer squash - peeled, seeded, and cut into 1-inch cubes

2 tablespoons olive oil

2 cloves garlic, minced

Sea salt Ground

Black pepper to taste

Directions:

Preheat your oven to 400 degrees F. Toss the squash with olive oil and garlic in a bowl. Season with sea salt and pepper. Layer the squash on a baking sheet. Roast in the oven until squash is tender for 28 minutes. Spicy

Fresh Herb-Roasted Summer Squash

Ingredients

1 large or 2 small summer squash, cut into quarters lengthways, seeds removed

olive oil, for drizzling

2 tbsp extra virgin olive oil

Sea salt

Freshly ground Black pepper

few sprigs fresh thyme, leaves only, plus

few sprigs fresh thyme, left whole

Directions:

Preheat your oven to 350 F. Layer the squash in a roasting pan with the cut-sides up. Drizzle with olive oil. Season with salt and freshly ground black pepper. Sprinkle the thyme leaves Roast in the preheated oven for 48 minutes, or until tender.

Roasted Red Cabbage and Carrots

Ingredients

1/4 cup Extra Virgin Olive Oil (you may need a bit more)

3 medium carrots, peeled and cut into 1 - 1-1/2 inch chunks

1/2 pound small red cabbage, outer leaves removed and halved

1 pound baby red potatoes, halved or quartered

1 large red onion, halved and cut into thick 1-inch pieces

1 pound (about 1-1/4 cup) sweet potatoes, peeled and cut into 1 1/2-inch thick slices

3/4 tablespoon dried oregano

3/4 tablespoon dried crushed rosemary

1 teaspoon dried thyme

1 teaspoon dried basil

Freshly cracked pepper and sea salt

Optional:

fresh herbs (such as thyme or parsley) to garnish with

Directions:

Preheat your oven to 400 degrees F. Layer all the prepared vegetables on the prepared pan Mix in the oregano, rosemary, thyme, and basil. Season with salt and pepper to taste Add the olive oil and toss together with all of the vegetable mixture. Roast in the middle rack for 35 to 40 minutes, flipping every 20 minutes

Slow Cooked Curried Lima Beans and Winter Squash

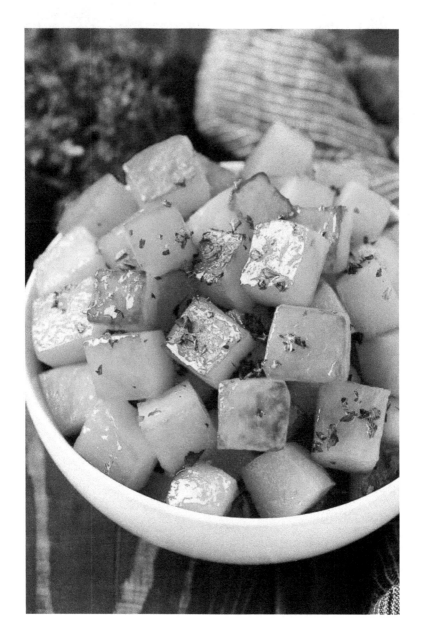

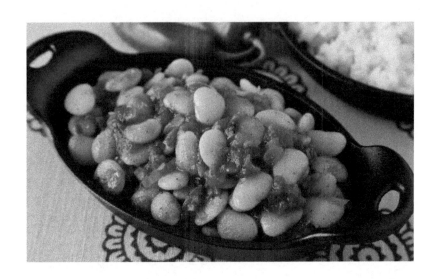

Ingredients

1 medium red onion chopped

5 garlic cloves minced

1 small winter squash peeled and chopped into bite sized pieces

1 green bell pepper chopped

3/4 cup red lentils

1 ,15 oz can lima beans, drained and rinsed

1 ,15 oz can tomato sauce

1 teaspoon freshly grated ginger

1 teaspoon turmeric

1 teaspoon cumin

1 teaspoon Spanish paprika

1/2 teaspoon cinnamon

1/2 teaspoon sea salt

Black pepper

3 cups vegetable broth to serve: cooked quinoa arugula coconut yogurt

Directions:

Combine all ingredients thoroughly in a slow cooker. Cook on high for 3 1/2 hours or 6 1/2 hours on low. To make it thicker, take out the cover an 1 hour before serving. Garnish with quinoa, arugula and non-dairy yogurt.

Macaroni with Mozzarella and Parmesan Cheese

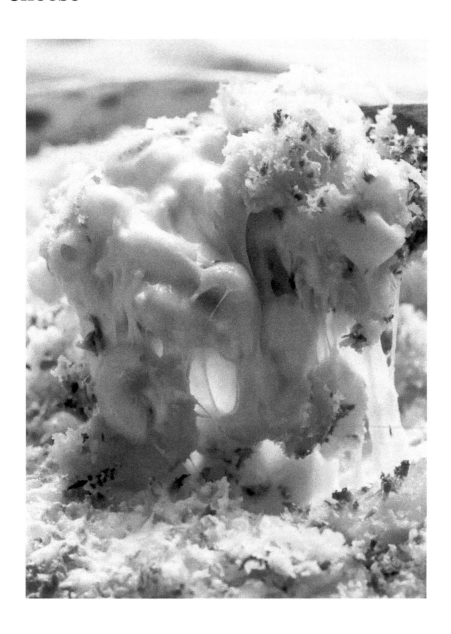

Ingredients

1 yellow onion, medium chopped

1 red bell pepper, chopped

15 ounce can fava beans, rinsed and drained

15 ounce can navy beans, rinsed and drained

28 ounce crushed tomatoes

3 ounces mozzarella

1 ounce grated parmesan

1 tsp. Italian seasoning

½ teaspoon salt 1

/8 teaspoon Black pepper

2 cups vegetable stock

8 ounces whole wheat elbow macaroni pasta uncooked

1 ½ cups Vegan Cheese (Tofu Based)

Garnishing ingredients:

chopped green onions for serving

Directions:

Put all of the ingredients except for pasta, vegan cheese, and garnishing ingredients in your slow cooker. Combine and cover. Cook on high heat for 4 hours or low heat for 7 hours.

Add the pasta and cooking on high heat for 18 minutes, or until pasta becomes al dente Add 1 cup of cheese and stir. Sprinkle with the remaining vegan cheese and garnishing ingredients

Spaghetti in Chimichurri Sauce

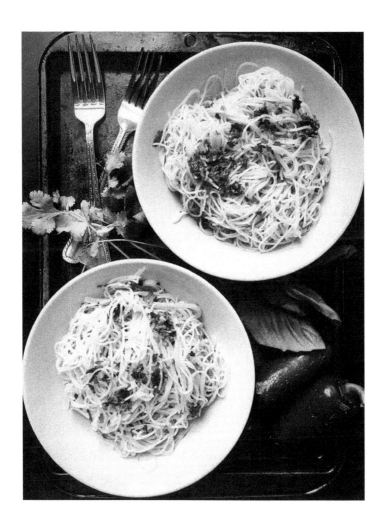

Ingredients

5 jalapeno peppers

1 red onion, chopped

15 ounce can pinto beans rinsed and drained

15 ounce can lima beans rinsed and drained

4 tbsp. chimichurri sauce

1/2 tsp. cayenne pepper

½ teaspoon salt

1/8 teaspoon black pepper

2 cups vegetable stock

8 ounces spaghetti uncooked

1 ½ cups Ricotta cheese

Garnishing ingredients:

chopped green onions for serving

Directions:

Put all of the ingredients except for pasta, vegan cheese, and garnishing ingredients in your slow cooker. Combine and cover. Cook on high heat for 4 hours or low heat for 7 hours. Add the pasta and cooking on high heat for 18 minutes, or until pasta becomes al dente Add 1 cup of cheese and stir. Sprinkle with the remaining vegan cheese and garnishing ingredients

Pappardelle Pasta and Parmesan Cheese

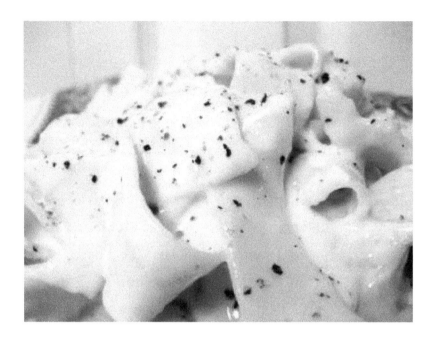

Ingredients

1 red onion, medium chopped

1 green bell pepper chopped

28 ounce crushed tomatoes

4 tbsp. cream cheese

1 tsp. herbs de Provence

½ teaspoon salt

1/8 teaspoon black pepper

2 cups vegetable stock

8 ounces pappardelle pasta uncooked

1 ½ cups grated parmesan cheese

Garnishing ingredients:

chopped green onions for serving

Directions:

Put all of the ingredients except for pasta, cream cheese, and garnishing ingredients in your slow cooker. Combine and cover. Cook on high heat for 4 hours or low heat for 7 hours. Add the pasta and cooking on high heat for 18 minutes, or until pasta becomes al dente Add 1 cup of parmesan cheese and stir. Sprinkle with the remaining parmesan cheese and garnishing ingredients

Pasta Shells with Beans and Mozzarella

Ingredients

1 yellow onion, medium chopped

1 red bell pepper, chopped

15 ounce can butterbeans, rinsed and drained

15 ounce can black beans , rinsed and drained

28 ounce crushed tomatoes

3 ounces mozzarella

1 tsp. Italian seasoning

½ teaspoon salt

1/8 teaspoon black pepper

2 cups vegetable stock

8 ounces pasta shells uncooked

1 ½ cups Parmesan Cheese

<u>Garnishing ingredients:</u>

chopped green onions for serving

Directions:

Put all of the ingredients except for pasta, mozarella cheese, and garnishing ingredients in your slow cooker. Combine and cover. Cook on high heat for 4 hours or low heat for 7 hours. Add the pasta and cooking on high heat for 18 minutes, or until pasta becomes al dente Add 1 cup of parmesan cheese and stir. Sprinkle with the remaining parmesan cheese and garnishing ingredients

Lightning Source UK Ltd.
Milton Keynes UK
UKHW020717270521
384465UK00005B/216

9 781802 695472